GARLIC FOR GOOD HEALTH

Why and How to Take Garlic

•

Safety and Efficacy of Garlic

•

Garlic and Disease Prevention

•

Different Types of Garlic Products

This UK edition published 1991.

ISBN 1-873492-02-2
published by

NUTRI-**HEALTHDATA LTD**

Milton Keynes, MK11 3HF, England.

This book does not intend to diagnose disease nor to provide specific medical advice. Its intention is solely to inform and educate. The author and publisher intend that readers will use the information presented in this book in cooperation with a medical or health professional.

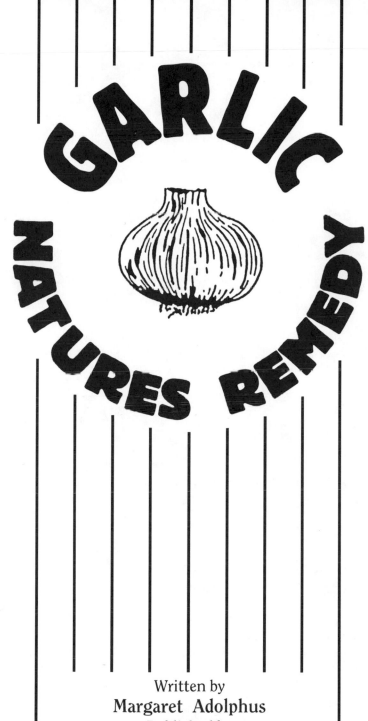

GARLIC
NATURES REMEDY

Written by
Margaret Adolphus
Published by
NUTRI-HEALTHDATA LTD

Table of Contents

CHAPTER ONE

Garlic: Spice Rack or Medicine Chest?

As Westerners, we are not accustomed to the kind of death from starvation that we see flashed across our television screens in news reports from Third World Countries. Indeed, we live amidst affluence. We expect to live long lives marked by good health. And we believe that if disease does strike, modern medicine will rush forward with a cure.

But that's not always the case – not even in the affluent West. Too many of us are dying prematurely. One in three will develop cancer. More than 120,000 die of heart disease every year. There are more than a million diabetics in the United Kingdom alone. And it is becoming increasingly clear that the under-funded National Health Service cannot effectively address the situation.

What is the answer? Perhaps the old adage says it best:
An ounce of prevention is worth a pound of cure.

One of the most effective forms of prevention is dietary. Medical science has soundly demonstrated that cancer, heart disease, stroke, and diabetes are caused at least in part by what we eat. High-fat foods loaded with salts or sugars are the culprits. The prevention may lie in foods that are low in fat and high in fibre and carbohydrates – fresh fruits, fresh vegetables and whole grains.

And then there are herbs: you might think of them as the dried bits of flavouring in the spice jars lining the door of your kitchen cupboard, but many of them also have a long history of medicinal use. A good example is garlic – a pungent spice, it has been used with success since ancient times as an effective medicine.

Garlic – often cooked, but sometimes raw – has been used in traditional Chinese medicine to treat conditions as diverse as angina pectoris, shigellosis, bronchitis, tuberculosis, appendicitis, malaria, boils, heart disease, tumours and various skin diseases.[1] Interestingly, the Chinese traditionally aged whole clove garlic in vinegar for two to three years to enhance its medicinal properties.[1]

As is often the case with herbal 'cures', many of the claims for garlic have proved to be myths. But others have proved legitimate – either through hundreds of years of effective use, or through careful scientific testing. In fact, nearly two thousand scientific papers reporting on garlic research have been published during the last two decades.[2]

What makes garlic an effective medicine?

The key to garlic's medicinal value is alliin, a unique sulphur-containing compound of garlic. Alliin is converted to allicin when garlic is crushed. Despite its strong smell however, allicin is extremely fragile. It reacts easily with other substances, and it's unstable: if allowed to stand at room temperature for a day, only 1 per cent of the allicin remains.[1]

The discovery of allicin in the 1950's was accompanied by great scientific excitement: because it had the power to kill cells in test tubes and petri dishes, allicin showed promise as an antibiotic. The promise was dashed however: allicin's instability gave it too short a life to be effective as an antibiotic. But there was an even more serious problem: allicin could not distinguish between harmful cells (such as bacteria) and harmless cells (such as ordinary human cells). It destroyed both.

Scientists went back to the laboratory in an attempt to determine which compounds in garlic did have medicinal value. Through careful scientific testing, researchers discovered the answer: two groups of sulphur compounds.

The first, the sulphur amino acids, include S-allyl cysteine and gamma-glutamyl-S-allyl cysteine. Besides being medicinally valuable, the sulphur amino acids are odourless.

The second group of medicinal sulphur compounds in garlic includes methyl-allyl sulphide and di-allyl sulphide.

Garlic: Used three ways

Garlic is traditionally used in three different ways. One is raw, whole-clove garlic; conventional garlic powders are made by drying raw whole-clove garlic. Unfortunately, raw garlic is less safe than cooked because of the dangerous side effects of allicin – cooking converts alliin to the more preferable sulphur compounds, including S-allyl cysteine. Traditional Chinese medicine called for cooked garlic rather than raw, whole-clove garlic.[1]

Another is garlic oil, which is obtained by steam distillation of garlic and is usually diluted with soyabean or other vegetable oils. But garlic oil consists of certain sulphur compounds that are, in fact, quite toxic. And since the sulphur compounds in garlic oil are volatile, they produce the pungent odour that causes bad breath.

Finally, aged garlic is preserved with methods that increase its nutritional and medicinal values. A centuries-old secret to enhancing garlic's medicinal properties was to preserve it – and the Chinese pickled whole-clove garlic in vinegar. Researchers in twentieth-century Japan discovered a similar method of 'aging' garlic: raw garlic is minced and preserved in large stainless steel tanks for twenty months before being extracted and concentrated.

Why is the aging process so beneficial?

During the aging process alliin and allicin are changed to water-soluble organo-sulphur compounds, such as S-allyl cysteine and S-allyl mercaptocysteine. In the process, the toxic potential of raw garlic is greatly reduced. The result? Aged garlic extract – which provides powerful medicinal benefits without toxic side effects.

CHAPTER TWO

Reducing the Risk of Heart Disease

Almost half the men and more than a fourth of the women who die between the ages of forty-five and fifty-four succumb to diseases of the heart and circulatory system. Heart disease is Britain's biggest killer. It is also the nation's most expensive illness.

Most who die of heart disease die because the arteries leading to the heart get clogged with fatty deposits. As a result, blood can't circulate effectively to the heart and part of the heart dies. When the same thing happens to the brain, a stroke results.

Science has established two major risk factors for heart disease. One is high blood pressure. The other is high levels of blood cholesterol, the fatty substance that deposits in the arteries. Blood cholesterol levels tend to increase with consumption of saturated fats (those from animal origins).

A special study of heart disease conducted by the Department of Health revealed that the British eat too many foods high in saturated fats. Government-issued dietary recommendations call for reducing dietary fat and increasing dietary fibre. Translated into simple terms, it means eating polyunsaturated margarine instead of butter. Eating fish and poultry rather than red meat. Eating low-fat cheeses – such as Edam, Brie, and cottage cheese – rather than high-fat cheese (such as Cheddar cheese). Using skimmed or low-fat milk instead of whole milk or cream.[3]

A separate study had fascinating results: Asians in Britain run a 50 per cent greater chance of suffering from heart disease than those who stayed in their native land – a trend that has increased in recent years. Why? Researchers believe it's because they have abandoned the tradition of eating garlic every day.

The garlic- cholesterol connection

The scientific results are in: garlic helps lower blood cholesterol levels.

Plenty of scientific proof backs up the notion that garlic can bring down cholesterol levels. One study, published in Nutrition Research,[4] used aged garlic extract over a period of six months. In the first part of the study, thirty-two people with high cholesterol were randomly divided into two groups. The first group was given four capsules daily of liquid aged garlic extract. The second was given a placebo (four capsules of a caramel-coloured liquid indistinguishable from aged garlic extract). Levels of blood lipids (fatty deposits) were measured each month during the study.

During the first two months of the study, there was no significant change among those taking the placebo. Not so with the aged garlic extract group however: their blood lipids actually rose during the first two months of the study. Discouraged researchers decided against abandoning the study when they learned that a similar phenomenon had occurred in an earlier study using garlic juice.[5]

By the end of the third month, lipids amongst those taking aged garlic extract had started to drop. By the end of six months, blood lipid levels had returned to normal in 65 per cent of the people who took aged garlic extract. There was no such drop among those taking the placebo.

What about the initial rise in blood lipids? Researchers believe that the garlic shifted lipids deposited in body tissues to the bloodstream, initially causing blood lipid levels to rise but eventually allowing the lipids to be excreted from the body.

In the second part of the study, researchers considered the impact of garlic on high and low-density lipoproteins. High-density lipoproteins (HDLs) carry excess cholesterol to the liver, where it decomposes; they protect against heart disease and stroke. Low-density lipoproteins (LDLs) carry cholesterol to the organs and tissues of the body; they contribute to the risk of heart disease and strokes.

When patients with high cholesterol levels took aged garlic extract for six months, what happened? The levels of HDLs (that protect against heart disease) steadily rose. The levels of LDLs (that contribute to heart disease) rose initially, but then steadily dropped.

Researchers concluded that aged garlic extract can significantly reduce dangerous levels of blood cholesterol. One reason why, they say, is simple: garlic inhibits the body from manufacturing its own cholesterol. (More than 70 per cent of the body's cholesterol is produced by the body itself.)[1] Apparently the sulphur compounds in garlic counteract the biological reaction that produces cholesterol and inhibit formation of one of the enzymes needed to produce cholesterol.[6]

Garlic packs additional benefits too: not only does it help reduce cholesterol, but studies have shown that garlic can reverse existing damage to arteries.

Garlic and blood clotting

Traditionally, Chinese practitioners relied on garlic to promote blood circulation and dissolve clots in blood vessels.

Blood can't circulate effectively if vessels are clogged with blood clots, just as traffic on a motorway slows to a crawl – or stops altogether – if the road is 'clogged' with stalled cars. Blood clots compromise circulation. In the worst possible scenario, a clot forms in one of the arteries leading to the heart (a coronary artery) – a condition called coronary thrombosis. The result? Myocardial infarction, or heart attack.

What part does garlic play?

To understand the beneficial role of garlic, it's important to understand how clots form. Blood clots are made up mostly of platelets (networks of small disc-shaped cells), fibrin (a mesh-like substance produced when blood coagulates), and trapped red blood cells. Several studies have shown that garlic interrupts the process by which platelets and fibrin work to form clots. Garlic and its compounds have also been shown to reduce fibrin formation and to break up existing fibrin.

The body depends on an intricate system of checks and balances to maintain perfect health. The process of blood clotting provides a perfect example. On the one hand, thromboxane (produced by the platelets) triggers clotting. On the other hand, prostacyclin (produced by cells lining the blood vessels) guards against clotting. An aqueous extract of garlic has recently been shown[8] to preserve the body's balance by inhibiting thromboxane but not prostacyclin production.

One garlic compound particularly effective against clotting is ajoene, a sulphur compound derived from allicin under certain conditions. Ajoene has been scientifically shown[7] to be as powerful as aspirin in preventing blood clots. It's important to realise that ajoene formation must occur at temperatures well above room temperature, so it is absent from raw or freeze-dried garlic.

Knowing this, you might be tempted to use garlic like you would a 'morning-after pill', continuing to eat a diet loaded with fatty foods and relying on garlic to undo the damage. Don't do it! Garlic has tremendous effects on the circulatory system when used as part of an overall strategy that combines garlic with a sensible, reduced-fat diet. The two together can lead to the greatest possible benefits from one of nature's best remedies.

CHAPTER THREE

Garlic: A Powerful Immune-Booster

Has anyone ever suggested that you wear a clove of garlic to stave off a cold?

You probably dismissed the notion as pure folklore. But wait a minute: garlic has been widely used in 'folk medicine' to relieve sore throat, to ease the common cold, and to prevent wound infection.

There's more to it than just folklore. For instance, physicians during World War One used garlic to prevent even massive battle wounds from becoming infected. During the early 1950's the Chinese successfully treated influenza symptoms with injections containing garlic extract. In the West, it was successfully used to prevent the common cold.[9]

As so often happens, the old 'folk remedies' are gradually being given credence in the scientific laboratory. Less than a decade ago, scientists worldwide became fascinated with traditional Chinese use of garlic, and the studies began in earnest.

In one, researchers at the University of New Mexico School of Medicine and the Albuquerque Veterans Administration Medical Centre[10] decided to test the anti-viral properties of garlic. In a test-tube experiment they used garlic to treat an influenza virus (influenza B/Lee/40), a herpes simplex virus (cause of the common cold sore), and the Coxsackie virus. The garlic was found effective against the influenza and herpes virus. (Tests were not conducted among human subjects.)

Viruses aren't the only organisms that produce disease: garlic has also been tested against bacteria, fungi, yeast, and other microorganisms. One study showed that garlic extract stifles the growth of fungi in the test tube.[11] Another showed that garlic powder stops the growth of *Candida albicans*, a common yeast.

Chances are good that you're familiar with *Candida albicans* – it's the culprit that causes vaginal 'yeast infections', characterised by itching, inflammation, and a white, odorous discharge. Candida inhabits the digestive tract, too, and is responsible for the white thrush infection common amongst infants and children.

How does garlic stop Candida growth? Several studies provide some answers. One[12] demonstrated that garlic prevents Candida from getting oxygen, thereby preventing its growth. Another study[13] using aged garlic extract showed that the garlic stimulated the body's inflammatory cells (those that fight infection) to produce substances that killed the Candida.

How garlic impacts the immune system

The immune system is the body's mainline defence – not only against minor irritations (such as the common cold), but against life-threatening diseases as well (such as cancer). In fact, the immune system features a powerful 'surveillance' system that seeks out and destroys defective or mutinous cells, such as cancer cells.[1]

That's what happens when the immune system is healthy. Unfortunately, a number of things can weaken the immune system. Your immunity can be compromised by poor diet, environmental pollution, stress and even the natural process of aging. Fortunately, there are also things that stimulate the immune system and one of them is garlic.

Garlic is rich in sulphydryl and polysulphide compounds. They sound complex but, simply stated, they promote activity of the immune system cells, especially the macrophages and the natural killer cells (important to the body's 'surveillance' system).

A number of studies have shown that garlic enhances the activity of the lymphocytes and the macrophages, immune cells that protect against disease either by producing antibodies or by attacking foreign invaders directly. One study showed that lymphocytes and macrophages were attracted to the site where garlic was injected; others studies have shown that garlic extract attracts immune cells.

A landmark experiment[14] conducted by Florida pathologist Tariq Abdullah tested the effect of garlic on natural killer cells. Dr Abdullah randomly divided volunteers into three groups. Over a three-week period one group took raw garlic, one group took aged garlic extract, and the third group (the control group) took no garlic at all. At the end of the three weeks, Dr Abdullah took blood samples from each volunteer and tested natural killer cells in the blood against tumour cells in test tubes.

The results were staggering. The natural killer cells of those who took raw garlic killed 139 per cent more tumour cells than those of the control group. And the natural killer cells of those who took aged garlic extract killed 159 per cent more tumour cells than those in the control group.

Another recent study[15] – though limited in size – showed that garlic may even have some benefit among victims of acquired immune deficiency syndrome (AIDS). Ten AIDS patients were given garlic supplements for twelve weeks. During the time they took garlic, the patients noticed improvement in a number of symptoms and the researchers noted improvement in the patients' natural killer cell activity and general immune function. Obviously, further research needs to be done among wider patient populations, but initial results seem promising.

Garlic and rheumatoid arthritis: What happens when the immune system goes awry

Sometimes, for reasons not completely understood, something goes wrong; instead of fighting foreign invaders, the immune system declares war against the body itself. The result are 'auto-immune' diseases. One of the most common is rheumatoid arthritis, characterised by inflammation of the joints and synovial membranes (those covering the ends of the bones).

A number of studies have shown that garlic can help relieve the pain and inflammation of rheumatoid arthritis. There may be several reasons. First, it curbs the activity of free radicals, which cause tissue damage. Garlic also moderates the body's production of eicosanoids, which cause inflammation.

Further research is needed to define the effect of garlic on rheumatoid arthritis. It obviously moderates production of eicosanoids – but could it in the process slightly suppress immune function, possibly affecting the body's ability to protect itself against infection? These are challenging questions for researchers and the seeds for meaningful future research.

CHAPTER FOUR

Garlic and Cancer

One in three people will develop cancer at some time in life; one in five will die from it. To date, scientists have not found a cure – partly because its causes are so varied. Cancer can develop when the body contacts a carcinogen, or cancer-causing substance – which can be anything from a virus to a powerful chemical. Researchers believe that most cancers are caused by environmental carcinogens, most notably tobacco smoke and dietary habits.[16]

While cancer itself was not recognised as a disease until this century, physicians have diagnosed and treated 'tumours' for thousands of years. Traditional Chinese practitioners successfully used a herbal formula containing garlic to treat their patients who suffered from tumours or cancers.

That traditional use of garlic – and the fact that garlic helps strengthen the immune system – has prompted contemporary researchers to consider its value against cancer. No one is ready to declare garlic a 'cure', but preliminary findings are exciting, and justify further research and testing.

One scientific study in China, conducted during the early 1970's showed that injection of a garlic extract had a slightly beneficial effect against cancers of the nose, throat, stomach and lymph. Another study, published in the well-respected Journal of Urology,[16a] found that garlic was slightly more effective in the treatment of bladder cancer than the BCG vaccine currently touted as the favoured treatment.

While everyone is interested in finding a cure for cancer, research emphasis has been on the prevention of cancer – and garlic is emerging as an important possibility in protecting against a number of cancers.

One of the most broad-scale studies was conducted among two large populations in the Shandong Province of China.[17] Researchers were fascinated by the fact that residents of Cangshan County enjoyed China's lowest death rate from stomach cancer – approximately three deaths per 100,000. Yet residents of nearby Qixia suffered thirteen times that death rate from stomach cancer – approximately forty deaths per 100,000. Detailed physical examination showed that the Cangshan residents had much lower concentrations of nitrates (precursors of carcinogens) in their gastric juices, and researchers set out to find why.

Complex dietary studies revealed the probable cause: the average resident of Cangshan County ate twenty grams of garlic a day. The people in Qixia rarely ate any.

The results of this and a number of other studies suggested to researchers that garlic may counteract the effect of carcinogens, thereby preventing the development of cancer. Ensuing studies have proved that many of the sulphur compounds in garlic (such as the allyl sulphides and polysulphides) can mitigate the effects of some of the most potent carcinogens known, including the benzo(a)pyrene found in cigarette smoke.[18]

One study tested several pure compounds of garlic and aged garlic extract[13] on bacteria that had been exposed to various carcinogens. The garlic inhibited, or at least minimised, the expected changes in genetic structure that normally occur after exposure to benzo(a)pyrene. Garlic had the same effect on aflatoxin B1, a powerful carcinogen that can contaminate peanuts, rice, cereal grains, corn, beans, and sweet potatoes and that is linked with cancer of the liver.

How does garlic block the action of carcinogens? The answer lies in DNA, the complex genetic material found in nearly every living organism. In order for chemical carcinogens to cause mutation, and therefore cancer, they must first bind the DNA molecules in the cell. Garlic can apparently prevent some carcinogens from binding to DNA.

Aflatoxin B1 (AFB1) provides a perfect example. In its natural form, AFB1 is not harmful. When it enters the body, however, various enzymes cause it to metabolise; the resulting products bind to DNA, and the problems begin. Fortunately, all AFB1 does not lead to cancer: in many cases other enzymes render it less toxic or make it water-soluble so it can be safely excreted from the body.

One study showed that garlic can prevent AFB1 from binding to DNA by studying the interaction between the body's enzymes and the carcinogen. Scientists incubated liver enzymes and AFB1; some were incubated with garlic compounds, while others were not. Researchers then closely examined what happened.

Study results showed that garlic packs a double punch. First, the ajoene, di-allyl sulphide, and aged garlic extract inhibited AFB1 from binding with the DNA. But that's not all: the aged garlic extract actually stimulated the cells to produce two enzymes (glucuronide and glutathione conjugates) that enabled excretion of the AFB1.

Researchers concluded from the study that garlic may have a promising preventive role against cancer in two ways. First, it may prevent carcinogens from binding to DNA to begin with. And, equally important, aged garlic extract may help the body eliminate carcinogens altogether.

CHAPTER FIVE

Garlic as a Pollution-Buster

Pollution isn't new on anyone's agenda. Every political party talks about it and all politicians claim to be 'green'. The myriad effects of pollution shout at us from the television screen and in the newspaper headlines. While we have become a people dedicated to convenience, a people wanting to get places faster and spend less effort on housework and cooking, we have begun to realise the terrible cost exacted by those conveniences.

Obviously, pollution is bad for the planet. But it's bad for the body too. For example, chemicals and heavy metals in the environment are responsible for a whole range of non-specific ailments, and are particularly devastating to people with weakened immune systems.

Garlic and heavy metals

You might think heavy metal pollution is something you don't need to worry about unless you work with heavy metals. How wrong you are! Heavy metals are all around us, and all of us are victim. Take a look at lead, for example: It's found in paint, in common batteries, and in the exhaust fumes of automobiles. Scientific testing has shown that we absorb one thousand times more lead than did our ancestors a century ago. Or what about mercury? It can cause nervous system damage and paralysis; at high enough concentrations, it kills. Yet it is used in dental fillings and is a common contaminant of the fish we eat.

That's where garlic comes in. Research has found that the sulphydryl compounds in garlic bind to heavy metals, rendering them harmless to the body. These compounds have particular protective effects against lead, mercury, and cadmium. And since aged garlic extract is so rich in sulphydryl compounds, it is especially protective against heavy metal pollution.

Specific studies have tested the effects of garlic in general and aged garlic extract in particular against heavy metals. In one recent study,[19] ten test tubes were each filled with a suspension of human blood cells. Researchers then put a heavy metal in each of eight test tubes – lead was added to two, mercury to two, copper to two, and aluminium to two. Two test tubes were left alone and were used as controls.

Scientists then added aged garlic extract to one of the tubes containing lead, one containing mercury, one containing copper, one containing aluminum, and one of the controls.

Microscopic examination showed the result. The red blood cells contaminated by heavy metal underwent 'lysis' – the membrane of the cell was ruptured or otherwise destroyed, and the contents of the cell escaped. Simply put, the cells were destroyed. In the test tubes containing aged garlic extract, however, lysis did not occur – even in the presence of heavy metal contamination. Researchers concluded that aged garlic extract protects red blood cells from heavy metal damage.

Garlic and free radicals

'Free radicals' isn't exactly a household term – and you may never have heard it before. But it's a phrase you should know about. Why? Because, left unchecked, free radicals can do untold damage to your body.

What exactly are 'free radicals'? Simply stated, they are molecules that carry an extra or unpaired electron.[1] That may not sound so bad, until you take a closer look. A molecule is the smallest complete unit of any chemical; it consists of a collection of atoms that are held together by positively and negatively charged particles (protons and electrons). When the electrons are paired, everything's fine. When you have one that isn't paired, it becomes highly reactive to the molecules that surround it.

Sometimes that's good. For example, free radicals are an important part of normal physiological processes, like digestion: free radicals help tear apart food and help convert food to energy (free radical activity produces extra oxygen). Free radicals are also used by the immune system as chemical 'weapons' to attack invaders.

But sometimes things get out of hand. There may be too many free radicals in the body, or their activity might be uncontrolled. That's when problems start. These wildly thrashing free radicals can generate excessive oxygen (or oxidation) and damage surrounding tissues, resulting in disease. A number of conditions such as cataracts, atherosclerosis, rheumatoid arthritis, Parkinson's disease, and even some cancers have been linked to free radical damage.

Where do we pick up the extra free radicals? There are a number of sources. One is excessive exposure to X-rays. Another is radioactive contamination. Still another is pollution – free radicals are generated from pesticides, industrial solvents, petrochemicals, chlorinated hydrocarbons, and other substances. So don't think your only risk is on the X-ray table. You're exposed to free radicals in your water, your food, and your air, as well as household solvents, cosmetics, drugs, cigarette smoke and even some toys. Unless you're totally isolated from your environment, you're exposed to plenty of free radicals.

Where can you get protection? From garlic!

Scientific comparisons between garlic-eating populations and those that eat little garlic show the difference. The garlic-eaters live longer and have lower cancer rates, suggesting that garlic slows the degenerative processes of the body.

Apparently aged garlic extract protects more effectively than other kinds of garlic against damage from free radicals and oxidation, probably because it is so rich in sulphydryl compounds. As a matter of fact, raw garlic and conventional garlic powders may actually have the opposite effect.

One study done at the University of California actually showed that eating too much raw garlic causes the red blood cells to be oxidised which can lead to anaemia.[1] Not so with aged garlic extract: studies show that aged garlic extract actually protects the haemoglobin from too much oxidation. (Haemoglobin is the substance in red blood cells that enables them to transport oxygen throughout the body.)

The protective benefits of aged garlic extract have been shown in a number of other studies, especially those examining the effects of free radicals. One of the most destructive effects of free radicals is activation of carbon tetrachloride in the liver. Two key constituents of aged garlic extract are so effective in preventing carbon tetrachloride formation that its manufacturer, Wakunaga Pharmaceutical Company, has applied for drug patents on both (S-allyl cysteine and S-allyl mercaptocysteine).

Protection against radiation

You probably associate radiation with atmospheric fallout from nuclear tests or accidents (such as the one that happened at Chernobyl). Those are obvious sources. But another source of radiation is the radon emissions from granite – something scientists consider to be a major hazard of our day. The result on the body can be devastating.

Several laboratory studies have shown that garlic and garlic extract can protect against the effects of radiation. In one such experiment,[20] scientists incubated human lymphocytes (the immune system's white blood cells) in cultures of living tissues that had been removed from the body. Some of these tissues were then infused with fresh garlic and some with aged garlic extract. Scientists then subjected the tissues to radiation.

What happened?

In the tissues not incubated with garlic, 75 per cent of the white blood cells died within seventy-two hours. In those incubated with fresh garlic, all the white blood cells died within about twenty-four hours. But in the tissues infused with aged garlic extract, the white blood cells did not die. In other words, the tissues were protected from the damaging results of radiation.

Researchers concluded from the study that while fresh garlic may actually have toxic effects, aged garlic extract may protect against radiation damage.

CHAPTER SIX

The Effectiveness of
Garlic Against Candida Albicans

You've undoubtedly heard of *Candida albicans* – it's the organism responsible for the common vaginal 'yeast infection' and the widely publicised 'yeast syndrome'. The syndrome, reported to plague millions of Westerners, is characterised by chronic fatigue, muscle weakness, depression, short-term memory loss, severe premenstrual syndrome, infertility, vaginitis, a variety of gastrointestinal problems, severe diarrhoea, skin irritations, asthma, and a host of food and environmental allergies.

Candida albicans is not a foreign invader: the body normally has controlled numbers of it, usually in the gastrointestinal and vaginal tracts. The problem occurs when Candida proliferates A number of factors may cause such proliferation, but one of the most common is the use of antibiotic medications. Antibiotics destroy 'friendly' bacteria in the body, allowing Candida to grow unchecked.

The results can be devastating – and unfortunately they can be very difficult to diagnose. Few physicians are familiar enough with Candida infection to be on the lookout for it; too often, patients with the troubling collection of Candida symptoms are misdiagnosed. Even worse, many are dismissed as hypochondriacs.

A recent article in the *Washington Post* refers to the 'long-standing debate in professional circles over the syndrome, which has little credibility in the mainstream medical community because it has no fixed definition and because research on its presumed causes and characteristics has not been published in the more prestigious medical journals'.[21]

A recent editorial in the prestigious *New England Journal of Medicine* acknowledged the controversy surrounding the syndrome. Penned by Dr. John Bennett of the National Institute of Allergy and Infectious Diseases, it stated that 'few illnesses have sparked as much hostility between the medical community and a segment of the lay public as the chronic candidiasis syndrome'. Bennett concluded that the controversy is bound to continue until 'additional scientifically sound studies' determine whether the syndrome actually exists.

Other researchers claim that the syndrome does indeed exist – and the public seems to agree. Tennessee allergist William G. Crook wrote a book called *The Yeast Connection* summarising his experience with patients – which sold three-quarters of a million copies. Dr. John Parks Trowbridge, whose pioneering work with Candida led to the best-selling book *The Yeast Syndrome*, claims that the 'yeast syndrome' is 'sweeping our industrialised world, but most people don't even know they have it'. Other researchers agree, claiming that more people are ill with Candida than medical experts have estimated.

And that's not the only problem: Candida has stubbornly resisted treatment. One of the anti-fungal drugs most commonly used to treat Candida infection, nystatin, was recently found no more effective than a placebo.[22] As a result, even those physicians who have recognised the existence of the yeast syndrome have often been frustrated in their attempts to treat it.

Raw garlic: Not an answer

In an effort to find an effective treatment for Candida infection, researchers turned to garlic. After all, garlic had been shown over thousands of years to be effective in treating a variety of infections caused by an entire range of microorganisms, including fungus.

Early experiments showed that garlic might indeed have promise: researchers crushed raw garlic, and used it in test tubes against both fungus and yeast. The results were what early researchers had hoped for – the raw garlic killed the yeast in the test tube.

But did the same thing hold true in the human body? No. Repeated experiments demonstrated that raw garlic did not have the same effects on yeast in the body as in the test tube.

Not only is raw garlic not effective against yeast infections, but it can cause a myriad of unpleasant side effects, too. As Dr. Robert I. Lin, Chairman of the First World Garlic Congress, pointed out, garlic's indiscriminate oxidative power can cause both gastrointestinal disorders and anaemia, as well as other toxic effects in the body.[1, 23]

Aged garlic extract and Candida

While researchers discovered that raw garlic didn't work against Candida, they found that aged garlic extract is extremely effective against the yeast-like organism. Shanghai Medical University neurologist Yan Cai did years of research showing that a compound, derived from aged garlic, called di-allyl trisulphide is effective against yeast infections. And, say researchers, it works without toxic side effects. Speaking at the recent First World Garlic

Congress, University of Texas, M.D. Anderson Cancer Centre researcher Osamu Imada pointed out that 'when garlic is aged, its toxicity is greatly reduced, and aged garlic extract is almost without toxicity'.

In one landmark study, researchers at Loma Linda University found that treatment with aged garlic extract helped removal of Candida cells from the blood stream. The research team, was led by microbiologist Benjamin S. Lau.[24]

Why is aged garlic extract so effective against Candida? There are probably several reasons why, say researchers. Leading researcher Mahomoud A. Ghannoum of the University of Kuwait reported to the First World Garlic Congress that certain constituents of garlic damage the outer membrane of the Candida organism, causing it to leak and reducing its ability to attach to other cells.

There may be another reason why, too: Dr. Lau and his colleagues tested immune response to Candida following treatment with aged garlic extract. Lau and his colleagues found that it enhanced the activity of the neutrophils and the macrophages, white blood cells that are essential in the body's immune response. After treatment with aged garlic extract, these cells were more aggressive and more effective in destroying Candida organisms.[25]

CHAPTER SEVEN

How Effective is Garlic?

You've read some pretty impressive stuff about garlic. And it's not just folklore. It's scientifically proven evidence that garlic is a powerful weapon in the battle against disease and degeneration. So why is it that your doctor always sends you out with a prescription for a chemical drug and not one for garlic?

The answer is a simple one: there's not enough information about garlic available to your doctor.

It's not good enough for your physician to pick up a book like this one and scan it for information about garlic. You see, every drug has to pass stringent tests for safety and efficacy before it can be listed in your doctor's copy of MIMS – the 'bible' of prescription drugs. The tests determine whether the drug is safe; what its active components are; how it is absorbed, distributed, metabolised, and excreted; and whether it has any toxic effects. Other tests must prove that the drug is effective and does what it purports to do.

All these standards must be determined by a variety of stringent tests on a large number of patients. That kind of testing simply has not been done on garlic – despite the considerable testing done by the Chinese and by Wakunaga Pharmaceutical Company.[1]

Based on the testing that has been done, we know a great deal about garlic.

How safe is garlic?

The safety of garlic is an issue that can't be determined in a single word: there are different types of garlic on the market and some are safer than others.[1]

While raw garlic does have some benefits, it is probably the type of garlic with greatest potential for toxic effects. Taken in large doses, it can cause burns of the mouth, oesophagus, and stomach; oxidation of red blood cells; anaemia, allergic reactions, contact dermatitis, lethargy, soft stools, and dehydration (a loss or deficiency of water in body tissues).[1]

Few tests have specifically determined the safety of garlic oil or garlic powder supplements. We do know that pure oil contains toxic substances but before marketing it is diluted with vegetable oils, which makes it less toxic.[1]

Tests conducted have shown that aged garlic extract, has the highest safety margin of any garlic product.[26]

Garlic: A drug or a nutritional supplement?

When considering the benefits of garlic, it's important to realise that no one should expect garlic to work as effectively as modern drugs. Nor should anyone attempt to use garlic as a treatment without consulting a qualified doctor.

The watchword with garlic, as with all other products on the market-place, is 'consumer beware'. You're likely to hear all kinds of claims about garlic. Be wary. Someone might claim, for example, that because garlic kills a certain bacteria in the test tube, it will obviously cure disease caused by the bacteria. That's not necessarily true. What happens in the test tube does not always happen when a substance is taken internally into the body.

To put it pointedly, don't use garlic as a drug. Do, however, use garlic as an extremely effective nutritional supplement. Used with a sensible diet, garlic as a nutritional supplement can help protect health and will reduce your risk of heart disease, cancer, and free radical damage. Obviously, you can purchase a nutritional supplement (such as garlic) without a doctor's prescription. But if you are being treated for any illness or disease, make sure you tell your doctor before you begin taking garlic or any other nutritional supplement.

But aren't nutritional supplements only 'second best'? What can nutritional supplements, like garlic, do?

Perhaps their greatest contribution lies in prevention. To understand why, you need to understand the disease process. Germs don't always cause disease. Disease only occurs in a 'susceptible host' – someone whose immune system has been weakened for some reason and in the presence of predisposing factors (such as environmental pollution). In other words, germs only cause disease when the conditions are prime for disease.

A nutritional supplement, such as garlic, works to keep conditions from being prime for disease. How? For one thing, it helps to strengthen the immune system. If the immune system is strong, germs can't get a foothold. For another thing, it may help overcome predisposing factors, such as environmental pollution. (You've already read the evidence that garlic can strengthen the body against pollution's effect.)

In that vein, garlic has attracted mounting attention from the world's scientific community, and there is growing interest in garlic research. Recently, the National Cancer Institute of the United States developed a $20.5 million programme to study the effects of medicinal plants, including garlic. Studies on garlic are being conducted in laboratories throughout the world and the results of those studies will give us even greater evidence of garlic's importance as a protector of health.

But you don't need to wait for the results of those studies. We already know enough to know that garlic is a valuable nutritional supplement. Used properly, it can be a safe and effective way to protect your health and reduce your risk of disease.

The bottom line? One of the best ways to protect your health is right under your nose! The First World Garlic Congress Chairman, Dr. Lin, concludes: 'Uniquely beneficial to modern man, garlic lowers the blood lipid levels, reduces the tendency of blood clotting, and may decrease cardiovascular risk. It also provides protection against free radicals, oxidation, and pollutants.'[27]

First World Congress on the Health Significance of Garlic and Garlic Constituents

(Preliminary summary published in International Clinical Nutrition Review, 11:1, 1991.)

The First World Congress on the Health Significance of Garlic and Garlic Constituents was held on August 28-30, 1990 at the Willard Hotel, Washington D.C., USA. The Congress was sponsored by Nutrition International Co. and co-sponsored by Pennsylvania State University and the U.S. Department of Agriculture. More than forty scientists from fourteen countries presented their recent research findings at the Congress.

The beneficial effects of aged garlic extract became the centre of the Congress. Twelve of the forty-six presentations were related to the efficacy of aged garlic extract. Moreover amongst many commercial products on the market, only aged garlic extract was used as a test material.

Dr. A.A. Qureshi and his colleagues, at the University of Wisconsin, reported a decrease of serum cholesterol levels and a reduction in platelet aggregation by aged garlic extract and S-allyl cysteine in a hypercholesterolic model. Since serum cholesterol and clot formation are well known as risk factors of heart disease, which is one of the leading causes of death throughout the world, the lowering of the serum cholesterol level and the inhibition of clot formation by aged garlic extract were good news for the prevention of heart disease.

A series of studies regarding cancer and garlic was the most exciting news at the Congress. A total of twelve studies were reported, in which seven studies were related to aged garlic extract against cancer. Aged garlic extract and organo-sulphur compounds in garlic inhibited carcinogenesis, such as oesophagus, colon, mammary, liver and shin tumour induced by chemical carcinogens. Aged garlic extract also inhibited the growth of urinary bladder tumour and malignant melanoma cells.

Free radicals and peroxidation were shown to relate to poisoning and radiation toxicity, geriatric disorders and aging. Three groups reported that aged garlic extract inhibited chemical-induced free radical and peroxide formation and decreased radiation toxicity.

Dr. Itakura, a senior researcher of Wakunaga Pharmaceutical Co. Ltd., in Japan, showed new constituents in garlic, including allixin, a new compound identified in aged garlic extract, which has an anti-tumour-promoting activity.

Dr. Imada, from the University of Texas, reported a toxicity study of garlic. Excess intake of raw garlic caused digestive tract disorders and anaemia; however, his study showed aged garlic extract has no undesirable effects. It was suggested that allicin contributed to the side effects of raw garlic.

Dr. Robert I. Lin, Chairman of the Congress stated that, 'standardization of garlic preparation is needed; however, alliin and allicin producing potential cannot be used as an index for standardization. Standard substances should be effective, safe and stable; moreover, allicin has not been adequately shown to provide health benefits'.

Further, this Congress made it clear that, allicin is highly unstable and toxic in high amounts.

Dr. Itakura stated, 'Since T. Wertheim isolated garlic oil in 1844, about two hundred compounds have been reported as the constituents of garlic. Even though many studies have been conducted on garlic, many more are needed to clarify which compounds cause the most effectiveness in garlic'.

REFERENCES

1. Garlic in Nutrition and Medicine. Robert I. Lin, 1989. (Available from Nutrition International Co., 6 Silverfern Drive, Irvine, CA 92715, USA.)

2. New Protective Roles of Selected Nutrients in Human Nutrition. G.A. Spiller and J. Scala, Alan R. Liss Publishers, 295-325, 1989; CRC Crit Rev Food Sci Nutr 22: 199-271, 22: 273-376, 23: 1-73, 1985; Lancet 335: 114-115, 1990.

3. For more information contact the British Heart Foundation, 102 Gloucester Place, London W1A 4DH; telephone, 071-935-0185.

4. Nutr Res 7: 139-149, 1987.

5. Am J Clin Nutr 34: 2100-03, 1981.

6. Atherosclerosis 64: 109, 1987.

7. J Am Chem Soc 108: 7045, 1986.

8. Prostaglandins Leucotrienes Med 25: 139, 1986.

9. Medical Monthly, March 1950.

10. Planta Medica 460, 1985.

11. Med Hypotheses 12: 227-37, 1983.

12. Antimicrob Agents Chemother 30: 499-501, 1986.

13. Intern Clin Nutr Rev 10: 423-29, 1990.

14. J Natl Med Asso 80: 439-45, 1988.

15. J Oncology 2: 52-53, 1989.

16. Nature 254: 589-96, 1977; J Natl Cancer Inst 66: 1193-1308, 1981; Cancer Res 34: 2425-35, 1974, 44: 5940-58, 1984; New Eng J Med 310: 633-8, 697-703, 1984.

16a. J of Urology 137: 359-362 , 1987.

17. Acta Nutr Sinica 4: 53-58, 1982.

18. Many studies have been published on this; for example, Carcinogenesis 8: 1155, 1987, 8: 487, 1987, 9: 131, 1988; Nutrition and Cancer 8: 211, 1986.

19. Intern Clin Nutr Rev 9: 27-31, 1989.

20. Ibid.

21. The Washington Post. Curt Suplee. 'Study Casts Doubt on Yeast Syndrome.' December 20, p. A4, 1990.

22. Ibid.

23. Abstracts of the First World Congress on the Health Significance of Garlic and Garlic Constituents. (Available from Nutrition International Co., 6 Silverfern Drive, Irvine CA 92715, USA.)

24. International Clinical Nutrition Review. 10:4, 423-429, 1990.

25. Garlic Research Update. Benjamin Lau. Odyssey Publishing Inc., p.6, 1991.

26. J Toxicol Sci 5: 91, 1980; 9: 77, 1984.

27. Garlic: A New Perspective. Robert I. Lin. 1987. (Available from Nutrition International Co., 6 Silverfern Drive, Irvine, CA 92715, USA.)

USEFUL ADDRESSES

The Garlic Research Bureau
PO Box 40
Bury St Edmunds
Suffolk
IP31 2SS

British Heart Foundation
102 Gloucester Place
London
W1A 4DH

For further information on
Aged Garlic Extract contact:

UK:
Quest Vitamins Ltd
Premier Trading Estate
Dartmouth Middleway
Birmingham B7 4AT

Malaysia:
Antah Pharma Sdn Bhd
3, Jalan 19/1
46710 Petaling Jaya
Selangor Darul Ehsan
Malaysia

Index